Beauty and Hair Dressing of 1912

By
Madam Qui-Vive
(Mrs. Helen Follet Jameson)

ADDITIONAL NOTES BY
TALIA FELIX
© 2015

BEAUTY AND HAIR DRESSING OF 1912

CHAPTER 1

The Woman Beautiful

There's an old saying that it is better to be good than to be beautiful, but so far as our investigations go, we know of no law that prohibits a woman from being both. Certainly a woman is happier if she looks well and if she is happy she sends out a certain influence of happiness. There's many a discouraged, morbid woman who needs nothing more than a new topknot or a Sunday frock to make her new and young again.

The woman question has made wonderful progress during the last few years in all lines, and it is safe to say that the first great change came about when woman confessed that she desired to be sweet to look upon and stated plainly and boldly that she was justified in taking to such harmless little artifices and subterfuges as might improve her appearance.

In the good old days – which were good evidently merely because they were old – the loving mother declared that she was very glad that her little baby was born plain. Ugliness and saintliness were supposed to be twins, and beauty and wickedness were boon companions. If a woman were beautiful it was taken for granted that she was also vain and emptyheaded. The idea is now turned inside out. If a woman is not pretty and fair to look upon, it is because in most cases she has disregarded the opportunities offered to make herself so, for it has been demonstrated time and again that most women are plain because they don't know how to be otherwise. They do not discover the great possibilities within themselves. It is certain that all of us have our plain and also our lovely days. Why not make all the days lovely if we can?

Why not always look our best?

The city woman has some advantages over the woman who lives in the small town. She has wonderful beauty shops in which she can receive various treatments. But she must also combat atmospheric dust, the effect of noise and traffic on her nerves, and the general wear and tear of city life. The small town woman has clear, fresh air, soft water and all of nature's delightful cosmetics. She should stay young longer and she should be able to preserve her hair, complexion and figure by means of simple inexpensive methods. This book was born with a mission. That mission is to take beauty suggestions to thousands of women. Beautiful women make beautiful homes and beautiful

BEAUTY AND HAIR DRESSING OF 1912

homes make a beautiful world. Hence, with the aid of this book, we may do some good to the universe.

The influence of beauty has been an immense power from the very beginning of human life. If we go back to Grecian legend and story we find it gemmed with exalted types of heroic womanhood, each and every one of whom attained her influence over the hearts and destinies of men through the power of beauty, and maintained it by intellectual and ethical force. Which shows us that beauty is of many kinds – spiritual and mental as well as physical.

Every woman not possessed with beauty longs to know how she can attain this magic power. From the time that she is old enough to recognize her own reflection in the mirror until Father Time touches her head with silver dust she seeks the ways and means of making herself more presentable. This yearning for good looks is not a vain and silly idea at all; it is born in women's souls, and the woman who denies the seriousness of her desire to keep young and lovely has false and unnatural ideas. She contradicts the perfectly human impulses of her own heart. The Lord put beauty everywhere – in the blue sky, the flowers of the earth, the dewdrops and the birds. Surely He did not mean that human folk should make of themselves mere ugly blots upon His beautiful landscape.

BEAUTY AND HAIR DRESSING OF 1912

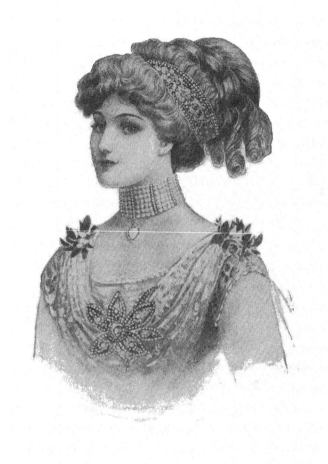

CHAPTER 2

The Care of Your Own Hair

Beauty ills are trifling or overwhelming, according to whom they belong – you or the woman next door. The bald headed man smiles sarcastically when he beholds a woman powdering her nose or sees her peering into a mirror, but when he passes his palm over his bald pate, the terrors and horrors of actual misery seize his heart as in a vise. He, like the woman with freckles and the lady with the fiddle string neck, would sell the shoes off his feet to be forever rid of his particular beauty ailment.

It's a hard matter to say just what kind of beauty trial is the hardest to bear, but there is one thing sure, and that is that a wealth of lovely hair can blot out and

BEAUTY AND HAIR DRESSING OF 1912

cover up many physical imperfections. A depleted halo is not as bad as an unsightly complexion, perhaps, but it gives one such a pinched, hungry, poverty stricken air that it certainly should be attended to and made to reform. The hair is much like the plant that stands in the living room window. Neglected it withers away and dies, but given a little thoughtful attention, it grows and flourishes, shoots out its branches and gives every evidence of gratitude. The hair responds quickly to care if given a certain amount of attention.

The study of the hair is very interesting. The root of the human hair, unlike that of plant or tree, will reproduce itself even after it has been completely plucked out. Hair is really a modification of the cuticle itself. The root is planted in the skin in an elongated shaft which projects from the root and the terminal point. There is a tiny bulbous like formation at the extreme point of the hair root.

All hairs are not planted evenly. Some are placed deeper in the cuticle, while many twist and turn, slant and curve, before reaching their own little cells, which are called the papilla and which produce the new hair when the old one is destroyed.

The quantity, quality and texture of the hair are governed by heredity, temperament and the general health. Nervous people seldom have thick, abundant hair. You remember the story of Sampson, of course, whose great strength was lost when his hair was cut. In nearly every case of falling hair the trouble is found to be defective circulation.[i] As long as the blood circulates with healthy vigor through the scalp, the hair will be thick and abundant.

BEAUTY AND HAIR DRESSING OF 1912

The first and greatest needs of the hair are cleanliness, friction and ventilation. Give your halo a sun bath once in a while and the silky strands will fairly laugh with happiness. For some reason there are many people who will not wash their heads often enough to keep the hair decently clean. If there is an inclination of dandruff, or if the hair is subjected to an unusual amount of dust, a shampoo every two weeks is an absolute necessity.[ii]

When the hair persistently suffers from loss of vitality it is usually from one or more of the following causes: Uncleanliness, lack of care, anxiety, worry, late hours, over-study want of exercise, or disease. Dyspepsia is responsible for many thinned out halos. The hair, being the most delicate of the body's formations, is the first to show that the body is not receiving sufficient nourishment. The use of harmful restoratives or dyes frequently causes the hair to become gray and broken. Too much care cannot be taken in the treatment of the hair and scalp.

The coloring matter of the hair is made up of the mineral ingredients in the pigment of the cells. These minerals change with age and health and vary greatly in individuals. Blond hair contains a large proportion of magnesia, while iron predominates in black hair, and sulphur rules supreme in brown or chestnut.[iii] When these minerals fail the hair becomes white. It is impossible to retard these changes by applying pomatums containing these minerals.

BEAUTY AND HAIR DRESSING OF 1912

CHAPTER 3

Suiting the Coiffure to the Face

Fairy stories are still doing business. Cinderella is not the only girl who was changed from a plain little sparrow into a beautiful bird of paradise. There's many a woman of the present day who has been so remodeled by means of a few hints given by the hairdresser, the gown maker and the milliner that she fears lest she might be obliged to go back to pigtails and pink gingham pinafores.

It has been said, "In the merciful scheme of nature there are no plain women." The woman with freckles and a pug nose will stand up and dispute this. However, it is a fact beyond dispute that if womankind would get an understanding of good taste, hygiene and rational living, the really plain, uninteresting woman would be a rare creature, something to be on exhibition at a

BEAUTY AND HAIR DRESSING OF 1912

museum and a subject for scientists to write about. The most beautiful woman that ever lived could make herself ugly by neglect, by wadding her hair in unbecoming coils, by topping these coils with a fright of a "bunnit" or by putting herself into impossible clothes.

BEAUTY AND HAIR DRESSING OF 1912

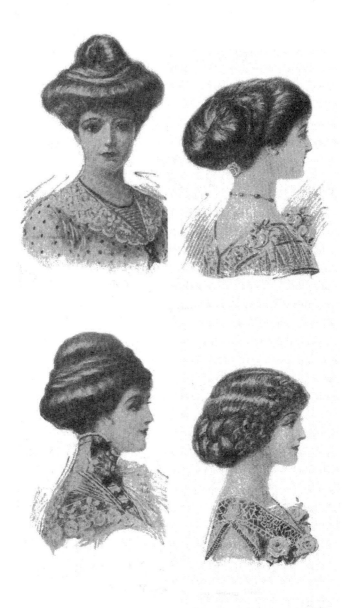

BEAUTY AND HAIR DRESSING OF 1912

To begin with the face: Every woman should understand both the defective and perfect lines. Her object is to hide both the imperfections and bring out the good parts. A proper arrangement of the hair is the main requirement.

Not one woman among five hundred can comb her hair straight back, sleek and severe, away from the face, and look any other way than unattractive. A few softening waves will not only make the hair seem thicker, but it will take away years from her age, and soften every bad feature of the face. Look at yourself in the mirror when you arise in the morning. Look again after you have given your tresses a fine "do." How about it? Changed? Well!

A mode of hair dressing which is tremendously becoming to one woman will be impossible to another. It all depends upon whether her chin is square or pointed, her eyes set high or low, whether her face is oval, thin, pudgy or beautifully curved. A careful, conscientious hairdresser, after ten minutes of judicious experimenting, will tell her exactly the kind of hair dress that she should wear.

The girl with a wedge shaped face must not wear her hair spread out over her ears. This only accentuates the triangular lines. With a peaked chin it is necessary to avoid broad effects above the brows. Wave the hair at the temples, draw it up to the top of the head in soft rolls. This gives the face a delicate oval outline.

The girl with the heavy square jaw and with the lower part of her face very broad must not wear her hair straight back so that the top of her hair is left flat. A straight fringe across the forehead is equally bad, for it helps make plain the straight cross lines of the lower part of the face. A woman with a broad square cut countenance must do her hair loosely and high and with breadth too, the coronet braid being exceptionally good for her style. Those of the sisterhood who have short chubby faces should follow the rule laid out for the girl with the broad, firm chin. A round, chubby face is improved by drawing the hair away from the face in a loose pompadour.

Upon the setting of the eyes depends whether the hair should be worn away from the forehead or drawn down over it. If the eyes are too near the top of the head the defect is exaggerated and emphasized by wearing the hair low on the forehead. If the forehead is broad and very high part of the wide expanse should be covered with the hair slightly waved. A bald forehead is becoming to very few women. The features are left harsh and plain. A few soft curls will give grace and beauty to almost any feminine countenance.

The girl with the long nose must never wear her hair parted in the middle or drawn far over her eyes like curtains. Neither must the pudgy faced girl arrange her locks after the Madonna fashion. This style is hopelessly unsuited to her face.

Very often the shape of the nose will determine the most suitable style of hair dressing. Many a woman will arrange a little bump of hirsute buns on the top of her head which matches the little bump of a nose on the front of her face. This is one great mistake. She looks decidedly "out of drawing."

There is only one argument against the pompadour, and that is the practice of "ratting" the hair underneath so that it will hold the waves out away from the head. This habit will invariably break and destroy the hair growth, the long strands gradually becoming ragged and of many lengths. A certain amount of roughening up with a comb will not prove fatal, but it is when the hair is left tangles most of the time that it becomes so ungroomed and assumes a generally unhealthy, unkempt appearance. At night let the pompadour lady comb and brush her tresses and arrange them in loose braids. This small attention is really due a respectable head of hair.

A small *inside pompadour* can be purchased that will do away entirely with "ratting." It is a splendid investment for the woman whose hair is thin at the temples.

BEAUTY AND HAIR DRESSING OF 1912

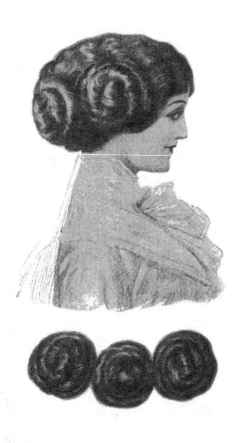

CHAPTER 4

The Use of False Hair Justified

We are happy to say that in these days of practical enlightenment the old time prejudice against false hair has entirely disappeared. Time was when the merest, tiniest switch was regarded with refrigerated suspicion and the woman who wore false hair lost the confidence of her sisters. At least some women entertained those opinions until their own locks gave way to age and despair, and then they changed their ideas. So it is with many matters in life. What we do and what some other woman does are entirely different affairs, based on an entirely different code of morals.

Every hairdresser will tell you that false hair can be arranged much more conveniently than one's own hair. The effect is usually better and certainly it can be kept clean much more conveniently. The woman with "hair

BEAUTY AND HAIR DRESSING OF 1912

enough to fill a bushel basket" is seldom able to dress it becomingly. The best she can do is to arrange the coils in flat circles around her head. She fears to "rat" her locks and the result is that they cling close to her head, giving a sleek, severe contour that is not half so charming as the loose fluffy effect of purchased "glory." It is a question whether a woman is lucky in having an immense quantity of hair. The woman who can afford a small amount of the purchased article can do up her hair in half the time and with half the trouble. This little booklet will give her careful directions for arranging the coiffure. Often a woman needs only a hint to transform a very ugly hair dressing into a structure of real loveliness.

It would be sad indeed if the prejudice against false hair still existed. It would mean that many a woman with a sweet, lovely face, would be doomed to appear in a state of semi-bald headed misery. That seems scarcely fair and certainly if nature deprives us of what is ours, none should blame us when we get the better of nature by replacing what is gone.

Each year shows wonderful improvement in designs in artificial hirsute decorations. Formerly switches were made with long stems and of ugly straight hair. Now the soft silky strands are so beautifully woven that the look even better than the real. The treatment of hair before it is given to the market tends to improve its appearance. It is glossy and of healthy appearance.

Just what style of hair should be worn must, of course, depend upon the character of the face and the outlines of the features. The great masses of curls that look very charming on a young girl are decidedly out

BEAUTY AND HAIR DRESSING OF 1912

of place on the dowager; while, on the other hand, the more stately middle aged coiffure is not suitable for the young.

The hair has such an endless supply of his wares that it is possible to secure a perfect match not only in color but in quality.

In the past many a woman dared not improve her appearance by wearing false hair because of her husband's opposition, but the men of today have fallen in line and the husband who says his wife shall not wear purchased beauty is numbered among those with ancient ideas. It is amusing to relate that there are husbands who do not know that their wives add to their hirsute glory by devious means and who greatly admire the attached decorations. Woman's advancement, which is without question the most important topic of the day, has done a great deal to help women to arrive at the conclusion that they are entitled to settle such small matters as these to their own satisfaction. No man stands in fear of his wife's opinion concerning the way he wears his hair. He does as he pleases. Surely if a woman enjoys any privilege at all it should be the privilege of deciding the small details of her personal appearance. She is taking that privilege nowadays. And the result is that women are young and pretty at the age that used to be the "shelving" period.

"It is my ambition to be the best looking girl my husband knows," says a wise wife, "and if I can keep his admiration by the addition of a few harmless little curls I'll have them if I have to cut down the grocery bill and skimp on shoes and clothing."

BEAUTY AND HAIR DRESSING OF 1912

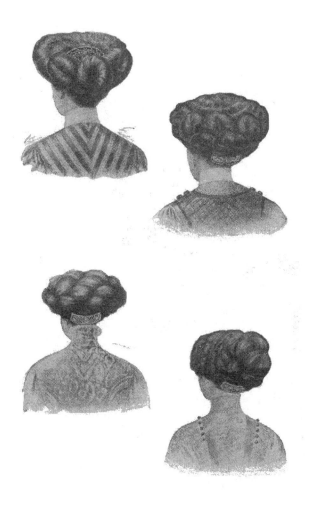

CHAPTER 5

Purity and Cleanliness of False Hair

It is impossible to conceive of any article that is cleaner or more sanitary than false hair. The methods used in the preparation and the cleansing of this product are absolutely thorough and antiseptic. In fact, it is very doubtful if any surgeon's instruments are subject to one-fourth the amount of boiling and cleansing to which human hair is submitted before it is finally made up for the trade. Thus the possibility of germs is eliminated and the result is that false hair is as clean, if not cleaner, than the hair on the head.

BEAUTY AND HAIR DRESSING OF 1912

The raw hair in its original state is received in assorted lengths just as it is cut from the head. The hair is first sorted into different lengths by means of a specially manufactured fine comb. These various lengths are then very carefully washed in boiling hot water, soap and strong chemicals, after which the hair is subjected to many hours of boiling. After this it is given three separate and distinct baths in peroxide of hydrogen.

After this operation the hair is dipped in strong cleansing acids which at the same time bring out the proper color. It is then tightly wound around sticks and boiled in a preparation of water and antiseptic fluids for at least six hours. The hair is then dried and once more carefully and thoroughly combed and is then ready to be made into any style desired; clean, fresh and pure in every detail.

From the above description of the process of purifying and cleansing false hair you can readily see that it is an absolute impossibility for any impurities or germs of any description to withstand treatment as thorough and radical as this.

A very ridiculous argument often used against false hair is the claim that the use of counterfeit locks impairs the health of the natural hair on the head. Many women will testify to having list their own hair through illness and that a fine, healthy, new crop has appeared owing to the becoming and convenient protection of a wig.

The rumors that appeared some time ago regarding the impurity of false hair were all thoroughly investigated by the health departments of various cities and found absolutely untrue in every detail.

BEAUTY AND HAIR DRESSING OF 1912

In conclusion we wish to say that as far as the purity and cleanliness of false hair is concerned there is absolutely no difference between the hair that grows on one's own head and the hair that is pinned on. It is absolutely certain that the beautiful effects produced by means of the false article cannot be accompanied without its use unless one's own hair is exceptionally long and thick.

BEAUTY AND HAIR DRESSING OF 1912

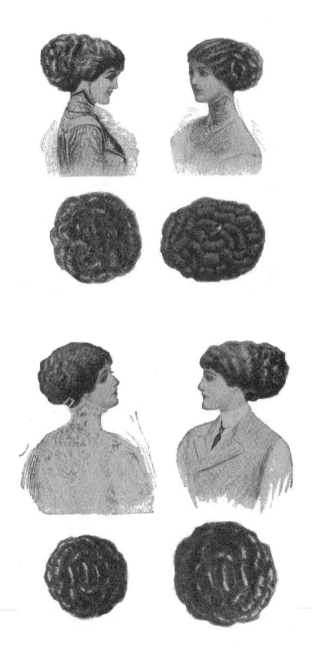

BEAUTY AND HAIR DRESSING OF 1912

CHAPTER 6

The Value of a Good Switch

For the woman who must invest in additional hirsute decoration the switch will always be the practical and economical selection. The possibilities of the switch are many and, without question, it has less of the "false" appearance than any other form of hair goods. A good switch will last for many years. It requires a little care and attention, that is all. It will wear away slightly, of course, but that must be expected. A woman will pay a good price for a hat or a gown and will take it for granted that its lasting qualities are limited. When she buys hair she expects it to last a lifetime. Its term of existence is not that long, naturally,

BEAUTY AND HAIR DRESSING OF 1912

but it will last until she feels that she has obtained many times the equivalent of her purchase price.

The very best hair will fade slightly, and that is why the sample from the head should always be cut close to the head to show the darkest shade.[iv] The end of the growing hair is always lighter and should not be matched. As a general rule the best sample is obtained by taking a clipping just back of the ear, an inch or two away from the hair line, or where the hair grows about the face.

Any woman can cut off a portion of her own hair and lay it away in the dark recesses of a dresser drawer and in six months she will scarcely know that it grew on her own head for the reason that it has faded. Without the natural oily nutriment the coloring matter weakens. To expect false hair to stay the exact same color for many years is to expect too much of nature itself. When false hair fades slightly it is not evidence that it was dyed hair.

By taking the sample from the darkest part of the hair the switch will change directly into the other shades. If all false hair has been cut for some time it will not change at all, but freshly cut hair is likely to fade a trifle. In making the selection of a color this matter should be taken into consideration.

A good switch of moderate length and weight can be arranged in a multitude of ways. It can be coiled or twisted, braided or draped flat across the head.

No switch is harmed by a little "ratting" or roughing, and that will make it appear more abundant and fluffier. It is a mistake to twist a switch into a tight knot and to pin on in harsh ugly lines. A softer effect is obtained by "ratting" the switch, each strand at a time, and then going over lightly with a brush to bring a neat surface. In that way a small braid can be made to appear much thicker and it will not lay down so close to the head.

A very simple way to make a coiffure for either the top of the head or the back is to tie each strand into a little knot, leaving it loose and soft and tucking the little ends underneath out of the way. This can be arranged on your dresser and it is no trick at all to pin it on the head.

The illustrations and directions appearing in this booklet furnish many varying styles that can be followed with no difficult whatever.

BEAUTY AND HAIR DRESSING OF 1912

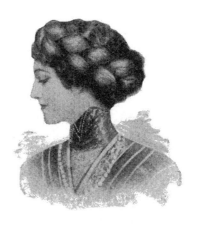

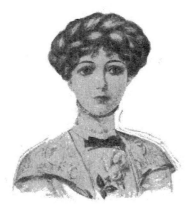

CHAPTER 7

Care and Cleaning of False Hair

The lasting qualities of a switch depend somewhat upon the care it receives. While it can be "ratted" to a certain extent, it should never be snarled or matted.

When the switch is removed it should be brushed briskly, arranged in a braid or coil and laid away in the dresser drawer.

It is not necessary to clean a switch or any other form of false hair oftener than once every two or three months. False locks do not gather dust as rapidly as growing hair for the reason that they have not the natural oil.

Hairdressers who understand the handling of "factory locks" can wash switches successfully and without matting the weave or stems, but it is safer for

BEAUTY AND HAIR DRESSING OF 1912

the inexperienced woman to cleanse hair by a dry process.

A simple method is to take equal parts of white corn meal and Fuller's earth, heating the mixture in the oven until it is quite hot. Place the hair in a glass jar and pour over it the warm meal and Fuller's earth, letting it remain there for an hour. Rub well between the hands, shake out, lay on a flat surface and brush thoroughly with a clean hair brush of stiff bristles. The hair will be soft and fine. A little brilliantine should be poured in the palm of the hand, the hair brush passed over the brilliantine and then applied to the switch.

It is best to keep a separate brush and comb for false hair.

Very fastidious women have a little box kept especially for their counterfeit frizzes and the box is lined with silk, under which sachet powder has been sprinkled. This imparts a sweet and lasting fragrance.

Curls and puffs can be dry cleaned, or they can be washed with melted soap and warm water. When they have dried on the radiator, pin them to an old cushion or any makeshift that you can devise. Take each curl separately, saturate with water and roll on large kid curlers. Let them stand over night or even several days. The longer they stand the better they will curl. Remove the kid curlers, comb out each curl, "rat" it slightly on the inside and roll up on the fingers, brushing the outside with a stiff brush just before the rolling. A suggestion of brilliantine on the brush will give the hair a gloss and will make the curls look fresher and more "alive."

Women who must resort to attached hair should not go about in the strong sunlight without a hat.

BEAUTY AND HAIR DRESSING OF 1912

Annexed tresses will fade in the strong light. One's own hair will do the same, for that matter. Women who play tennis and golf, who go almost through a summer without wearing a hat, always find their hair bleached several shades lighter by the time autumn arrives.

BEAUTY AND HAIR DRESSING OF 1912

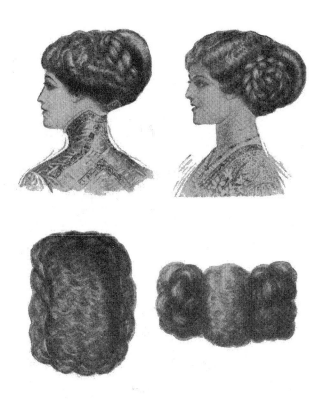

CHAPTER 8

Pompadours and Transformations

To very few women is a sleek, flat coiffure becoming. Straight, severe lines bring out every turkey track and wrinkle, and exaggerate every facial defect. If the nose is long, the flat hair dressing is particularly trying. The softer the arrangement of the hair the more fullness given to the coiffure, the less prominent will appear blemishes of the complexion or marks of age. Many a woman's appearance has become ten or fifteen years more youthful by the use of the necessary hirsute equipment to make her hair appear thicker and more luxuriant.

Especially necessary, to almost every face, is fullness at the side of the head and behind the ears. Fullness at the back always gives a better shape to the head.

BEAUTY AND HAIR DRESSING OF 1912

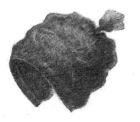

When the hair is very thin, scanty and practically unmanageable, there are two means of imparting an appearance of abundance. One means is the inside pompadour which is worn under the natural hair, and the other is the outside transformation which covers the natural hair. If the hair is very short and wispy and not thick enough to fairly cover the pompadour, the transformation is more desirable.

The inside pompadour may extend entirely around the head, or it may be placed merely in the front or at the back, found more satisfactory, as it can be fitted perfectly to the head and will stay in place better. The present styles in hair dressing really call for the all around pompadour, as there is a return to the extended effect.

Many women fear that they cannot manage these convenient little contrivances, but with a few directions and a little experimenting it is no trick at all, and the results are worth the effort.

The proper procedure is to comb one's own hair forward, that is, the front hair hangs down over the face and the side hair at the sides and the back hair over the shoulders. This leaves the top of the head smooth and plain. The pompadour, which is really a circular fringe, is placed on the head like a halo. It is pinned securely at the back, at the front and at either side. The pompadour is then "ratted" by combing the wrong

BEAUTY AND HAIR DRESSING OF 1912

way. This makes it thicker and helps it to stay in place properly. First a portion of the front hair is picked up, arranged away from the face and the ends pinned on the top of the head. Each side portion is treated in the same manner and finally the back hair is put in place. After the hair is all up a stiff brush should be used to give a neat surface and a trim appearance. If a hair net is used, such a hair dressing will stay in place perfectly for many hours.

If it is best to part the hair in the middle, it can be done, the circular pompadour being unhooked and each end coming just to the parting, or it can be united with a little black thread that will not show at all.

There are many advantages in a pompadour. It not only shapes the head properly, but it saves one's own hair from "ratting" and gives a good, firm, solid foundation for puffs, braids or curls. The hair can be waved or it can be worn plain. The ordinary kid curlers, worn at night, will give the hair a big loose wave and will look very well, especially if the hair is brushed the next morning. Brushing the hair after curling is always desirable as it causes the waves to fall into continuous lines, looking more natural and doing away with the fuzzy, kinky appearance.

The pompadour should match the natural hair perfectly. Then if the hair is thin and the pompadour shows, there is no distinction between the real hair and the counterfeit. The effect of the inside pompadour is neat and becoming to every face. It makes the full face look less plump and the thin face less thin. It is like the physical culture[v] exercises that work both ways – the same ones will develop and reduce. The truth is, it merely brings about a normal condition.

BEAUTY AND HAIR DRESSING OF 1912

The transformation is a ventilated piece, made with a foundation of net that fits the outline of the face. One's own hair can be entirely hidden or it can be drawn over the transformation at the temples. Transformations are made with or without a part and with or without bangs. They positively cannot be detected from the natural arrangement.

BEAUTY AND HAIR DRESSING OF 1912

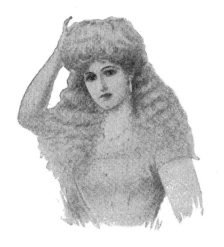

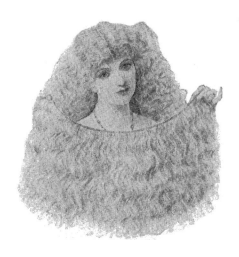

BEAUTY AND HAIR DRESSING OF 1912

CHAPTER 9

How to Wear a Wig

The sentiment against false hair is like everything else – it changes as the need for it approaches. False hair may be regarded as an affliction when worn by another woman, but it is the very life of one's soul when it covers one's own abbreviated halo.

The woman who sneers at wigs today may live to wear a wig tomorrow.

However, the wigmakers' art has progressed wonderfully the last few years. The work is done so skillfully and cleverly and the hair lines are so carefully concealed that many a wig will easily pass as a genuine head of hair. Without question, the woman who is prematurely gray and whose locks are scanty finds the wig of dark, natural hair a great blessing. If she is employed, it sometimes means that her very existence depends upon her appearance. In this age of youth,

BEAUTY AND HAIR DRESSING OF 1912

vitality, ambition and energy, it is absolutely necessary to appear young.

When ordering a wig, the most careful measurements are required, as every wig, to be satisfactory, must be made to order. It will be necessary to have the circumference of the head, the distance from forehead to the back of the neck, the measurement from ear to ear across the forehead and from temple to temple around back.

Wigs are made on a foundation of silk netting and are braced with tiny stays that give them shape. With great care every individual hair is drawn through this ventilated fabric with a fine crochet needle. It is not advisable for the customer to endeavor to clean a wig herself. This should be done by one who understands the proper treatment of wigs and usually the hair is given a "water wave" to make it fluffy and natural looking.

As wigs are not made light and ventilated, they have no bad effect whatever on the hair growth. There is very little weight to them. A wig is not only an aid to women's appearance, but it is a protection and health help. It is natural that the head should be covered. Mother Nature figured out that matter long, long ago. If we are deprived of our hair through illness, accident or age, it is essential that some covering should take its place.

The word "wig" has lost its ugly sound these last few years. Peek into the window of a fashionable hair goods store as you will envy the wax ladies who look smilingly at you. Their neatly waved tresses are not only correct but they are youthful and beautiful.

BEAUTY AND HAIR DRESSING OF 1912

Before putting on a wig, one's own hair should be brushed well and laid flat. If the hair is long enough to braid, it should be arranged in two plaits and these plaits wound about the head. Then a band of thin muslin is pinned snug and tight about the head. This gives a foundation and anchorage for the hair piece which can be made more secure with hairpins. Sometimes it is not necessary to wear the band, but most women who wear wigs feel more comfortable and more secure with a safe, sure bandage.

BEAUTY AND HAIR DRESSING OF 1912

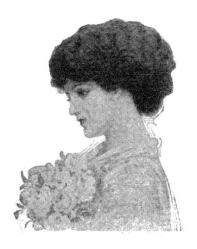

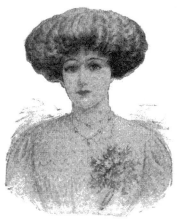

CHAPTER 10

Shampooing the Hair

Just how often the hair should be thoroughly shampooed depends upon the condition of the hair and the condition under which the individual exists. The school teacher, exposed to a cloud of chalk dust and the atmospheric soil of the schoolroom where many small feet are tramping about, will find the fortnightly shampoo a necessity, while the little home woman will only need to cleanse her hair once a month or even less frequently.

When dandruff forms on the scalp or when the hair is naturally oily, shampooing should be much more frequent than when the scalp is in normal condition or the hair is dry and wiry. Dry hair will not endure too much scrubbing. If given too much soap and water it will become brittle and will break easily. For very dry hair some good oily substance should be rubbed into the scalp occasionally or a first class proprietary hair tonic used. While oily hair is unmanageable and stringy it is usually much healthier than hair that is excessively dry.

When shampooing the hair, the soap should be dissolved.[vi] Never rub the bar directly on the head. Small particles of soap will be retained which the most thorough rinsing cannot take away. The hair should be wet before the soap is applied. The proper process follows:

Fill a washbowl with warm water. Hold the head over the bowl and with hands or a cup, throw the water over the head, wetting the hair thoroughly. Pour on some of the liquid soap, rubbing it in briskly. Do not be afraid of tangling or snarling the hair. The soap must be well rubbed in or the results will not be satisfactory. Keep on adding soap and throwing the water over the head until there is a rich live suds that has gone into every little corner and recess.

Rinse the hair well with warm water and follow with a second shampoo. In almost every case of the unsuccessful shampoo, it is because the hair has had only one soaping or because the rinsing has not been complete.

With a bowl of fresh water and with more soap, repeat the first process. Rub the scalp well with the finger ends, so as to dislodge all the dandruff. Pour some of the soap on the long hair. It needs attention quite as much if not more than the hair that is close to the head. The final rinsing should be continued until the strands are soft and silky. Experienced hair

BEAUTY AND HAIR DRESSING OF 1912

shampooers know immediately by the feel of the hair whether or not it is absolutely clean. If there is the slightest stickiness, if each hair does not stand by itself, the shampoo is not a success.

Running water is always better than water splashed up from the bowl. If one has a bath tub and spray with a rubber hose attached[vii], the problem of rinsing the hair is easily solved and the hair can be thoroughly cleansed of every particle of soap suds.

Wrap the head tightly with a hot towel, and pat until most of the water is absorbed. Shake out the hair and massage the scalp with the finger ends, wiping the long hair with warm towels. The hair should never be left to dry without friction. Such neglect will destroy the hair roots and prove destructive to the growth.[viii] The hair should not be groomed at all until nearly dry if you would have it fluffy and silky. Use the brush first, dividing the hair into sections. Then comb carefully.

The human hair is of such delicate structure that it should be given the most delicate and painstaking care. It will reward its owner by smiling up and looking fine. The hair has its seasons of health and illness, like other parts of the body. When it is shaggy, unmanageable and lifeless it is because it is not having proper attention. Brushing the hair for five minutes every night will give ventilation to the hair and exercise the scalp and will be helpful in every way.[ix] The rubbing in of a good tonic once or twice a week will prolong one's hair for many years.[x]

CHAPTER II

Proper Use of Powder and Rouge

The New York Medical Journal, the most dignified and conservative medical journal in the United States, endorses the use of pure cosmetics. The powder puff and the rouge pot are acknowledged as useful hygienic accessories. Following is a brief quotation of the article to which we refer:

"The use of face creams and makeups is universal and the moral aspect of the question is becoming settled. Our women now fearlessly and scientifically handle the complexion brush, the face cream, and the powder puff. Why is the face of a country woman sixty years old faded and wrinkled, while the face of a city woman of the same age frequently is smooth and

BEAUTY AND HAIR DRESSING OF 1912

beautiful? One account of protection against the elements. The city woman has been using her cream and powder for forty years and has yet to experience any deleterious effects.

The idea that the faces of actresses are old looking off the stage is pure superstition. Many an actress courted of our fathers has a complexion the envy of our daughters. These are things the physicians should know and not be afraid to say."

It is not an uncommon matter to hear a woman say: "I have never used powder in my life." It usually happens that the woman's complexion would appear to better advantage if it were powdered. The statement she makes is usually orated in a voice significant of great virtue and self satisfaction. Powder protects the skin from atmospheric dust and also from sun and wind. Good materials can be put in powder form as well as in creams or skin foods.[xi] There is no earthly reason why a woman should shun face powder as if it were poison.

The woman who keeps youthful and dainty never feels presentable without a bit of powder. It takes away the shine and the starched look and puts in its place a soft velvety surface, clean and pleasant, and gives an appearance of perfect grooming.[xii]

Excessive pallor is significant of ill health or drooping spirits and a touch of rouge on pale cheeks will not only make the chalky, wan face brighten up, but it will have a certain effect upon one's mental state. The woman who looks into her mirror and sees the reflection of bright eyes and rosy cheeks must certainly feel happier than the one who gazes upon the mirrored outlines of a pale, white faced, forlorn looking lady.[xiii]

BEAUTY AND HAIR DRESSING OF 1912

Powder should never be applied without a foundation of cream. Special greaseless creams are manufactured for the use of those who have oily skins.[xiv] This cosmetic vanishes as it is rubbed into the skin and just enough of it remains on the surface to hold the powder tight. When rouge is used it should be put on after the cream, and the powder is fluffed on afterward.

Powder should not be scattered about the face, but should be rubbed in thoroughly. The idea that it will clog the pores is nonsense. Many a mother who dusts the entire body of her infant with powder fears to put powder on her face. Life is certainly filled with many absurdities, and custom creates strange inconsistencies.

While too much rouge is always to be deplored – for the world has little use for the "painted lady" – a tiny touch of color will be found becoming. You doubtless know personally dozens of women of high social standing who have used cosmetics, rouge and powder all their lives and not one of them has any but the most exquisite and youthful complexions. To scare away wrinkles and give Father Time the laugh, the complexion should be given generously of some good skin nourishing oily cosmetic. Continual bathing of the face robs it of the natural oils and their equivalent is supplied by cold creams and skin foods.

It is best to remove powder and rouge with a bit of cold cream, although pure soap and water will do the work as well, and the cream can be rubbed in afterward.

CHAPTER 12

Retain a Youthful Appearance

THESE HINTS MAY HELP YOU

Anger, irritability, nervousness, petulance, sneers – these are all items that are only too quickly registered upon the note book of the human face. Avoid them. The only lines that are sweet to look upon are the little laughing wrinkles that sometimes come to the girl who is as brimful of smiles as a May morning. They don't make her look older – not a day – for they were caused by happiness and cheerfulness, and not by acidity of temperament or petulant thoughts. No skin food made by earthly powers will erase lines that are being made more indelible every time something goes wrong. There is no use wasting time in the hopes of smoothing out the furrows in your brow if you are a fretter.

BEAUTY AND HAIR DRESSING OF 1912

Whenever you find your heart strings sizzling over an injury, imaginary or otherwise, remember those delightful lines by Shakespeare. Katherine spoke them after she had been tamed:

"A woman moved is like a fountain troubled –
Muddy, ill-seeming, thick, bereft of beauty."

Next to a careful diet, the daily bath, regular exercise in the open air and cheerfulness of mind and heart, there is nothing so excellent in the beautifying line as a facial massage. This is especially so when the outer layer of skin has become too loose for the under one, like a bodice with a lining too snug. The outside material is sure to fold.[xv] Massage revives the under skin and sends the muscles about their business, instead of allowing them to become lazy and torpid. The bloom comes to the surface, making a pretty glow of pink, and the complexion takes on a new life, like a plant out in the showers and sunshine and given half a chance to be happy.

The one difficulty with home treatment is the fact that improper massage movements can cause a world of trouble. Keep in mind that when one trouble is being cured another must not be created. Therein lies the secret. The outer skin must not be stretched or allowed to fall into fine lines.

ONE MINUTE DIRECTIONS FOR FACIAL MASSAGE

Before beginning massage, the face should be washed well with warm water and a little castile soap. Powder and dust should not be kneaded into the pores of the skin. The wrinkle worried lady is seated in a

BEAUTY AND HAIR DRESSING OF 1912

reclining chair and the operator stands directly behind her. There is no chance of a doubt that the same results cannot be had from self treatment and for that reason I would advise seekers after beauty to help each other. "You smooth out my furrows and I'll rub out your crow's feet." Some of the movements can be done nicely by oneself, but others, like massaging the neck, must be done by someone else.

An ordinary cold cream is not suitable for massage, as body and firmness are needed. A massage cream is heavier and better.

KNEADING THE FACE

After the cheeks, forehead, chin and nose are carefully anointed with the skin food, the kneading should begin. It is almost impossible to describe this movement, as it is not merely a rubbing round and round in small circles, but an inward movement as well. Remember that the muscles close to the bone must be revived and exercised and that kneading does not mean a brisk pummeling of the skin alone. The circles should be small, but as the fingers sweep back to the starting point they must sink well into the flesh. We all know that the skin is constantly undergoing a process of decay and renovation. The muscles follow the same plan. The tiny cells of which the muscles are composed are continually being repaired. As the worn out particles are rejected the new fiber is created. Does it not stand to reason that massage will facilitate this process, make the flesh firm, and restore vigor to the muscles? This simple kneading movement is splendid for this purpose. If the circulation is defective the tissues soon become flabby, and a finely lined face is the result.

LINES ACROSS THE FOREHEAD

There are any number of forms of massage which are used for lines across the brow. The kneading motion described above is the first one used. The next movement is a difficult one to learn, but it can be mastered if one perseveres, and is the most effective massage movement that has ever been tried. The four fingers of each hand are placed so that a fold running crosswise the wrinkle is picked up. While the fingers of the left had push their way slowly across the forehead the fingers of the right rub up and down like a smoothing iron. As the hands make their way from one side of the forehead to the other the little fold goes too. It is never allowed to disappear. When kneading, have the general direction upward and outward. The surgical operation for this blemish is merely that of making incisions in the flesh on the temples under the hair, drawing the skin taut and sewing up a little tuck. Nothing could be less effective. Even if the wrinkles are gone for a while they soon return, as the main trouble, impoverished tissues and flabby muscles, is in nowise banished. When wrinkles are deep they must be raised up and gently ironed with the tips of the fingers. You can make no possible mistake if you follow these directions. See to it that enough skin food is applied so that the tender cuticle will not be bruised.

LINES BETWEEN THE EYES

Always have the muscles relaxed during treatment. These small lines running like accordion plaits between

BEAUTY AND HAIR DRESSING OF 1912

the eyes should be subjected to much the same treatment as that referred to above for lines in the forehead. The kneading must be upward toward the hair. The experienced masseuse picks up a little fold of flesh and rubs it between her finger tips until the line becomes too discouraged to care to exist. A simple and very good motion used for these fretting furrows is to pick up the tissues so the fold will be lengthwise of the line, then rub the crease with the finger tip, the thumb forming the ironing board and the finger the iron.

LINES AROUND THE EYES

Crow's feet or turkey tracks. No matter what the name, they're just as horrible. The flesh is held firm with the fingers of one hand, while the lines are wiped out of existence by a gentle, firm kneading with the first finger of the right hand. Like many other movements in massage, this is one that the little homebody can give herself with the best success imaginable. Another movement is to place the second finger of each hand on each side of the nose directly on the eyelid. The fingers then sweep out toward the ears, just a little beyond the eyes, and come back under the eyes to the starting point. You will notice that on the return trip the fingers rub the crow's feet the wrong way. It is the most effective treatment. With no other knowledge of massage than the understanding of these few movements any woman should be able to make the turkey tracks disappear.

LINES FROM NOSE TO MOUTH

These lines, like others, should first be treated to a little kneading, as described in the beginning of these directions for massage. Then the flesh is picked up, first in one place and then in another. The flesh is not rolled, for that destroys the tissues and reduces the fatty cushions, but it is picked up quickly, given a little rub with the tip of the finger and sent about its business, while the next section of the line is tackled. The patting treatments must be firm but gentle. The blood is sent tingling through the veins, and the cheeks get into a healthy, wholesome glow. When massaging oneself the fingers, of course, will point upward. Patting is particularly good when the flesh is soft and flabby and the complexion dull and lifeless. If the girl who wants rosy cheeks will try this occasionally she won't be fretting her life away because there aren't any roses where roses should be.

FOR HOLLOW CHEEKS

Before giving directions for treatment for hollow cheeks, let me say that a nutritious diet, together with outdoor life, but without too much exercise, will assist matter greatly. Sometimes a good fattening tonic is advisable, particularly if one is very thin or not strong. It is a difficult matter to put evidences of health in the face when health does not exist in the body. A woman who is troubled with indigestion of any sort need not expect that anything in the line of massage or cosmetics is going to accomplish any astonishing good. It is more than can be expected. Hollow cheeks are often a sign of malnutrition, although not always. There is no chance for an argument concerning the splendid results of massage treatment for this worry. The wall of the cheek is formed by the trumpeter's muscle, and it is when this becomes relaxed and flaccid that the glands shrink and the tissues emaciate. Manipulation forces blood through the muscles and they are thus strengthened and the tissues rebuilt. The muscle formation is not rolled between the fingers. The flesh is merely picked up quickly, first in one place and then in another. This is another movement one can do oneself almost as well as can the professional operator.

CHAPTER 13

The Care of the Hands

"God took his softest clay and his purest colors and made a fragile jewel, mysterious and caressing – the finger of woman; then he fell asleep. The devil awoke, and at the end of that rosy finger put – a nail."
–Victor Hugo.

In a woman's hand one sees the great possibilities of beautifying. It is the same with her hair, her complexion, her figure; for the hand responds no more quickly than these other parts of this most wonderful of all mechanical contrivances – the human body.

The very worst pair of hands in the world can be made beautiful, be they not deformed in any way, and in a very brief time, too. A little care, a little attention, a little thought – that is all.

BEAUTY AND HAIR DRESSING OF 1912

A woman's hand is such a beautiful thing – soft, dainty, of delicate lines and caressing touch. We might well be proud of these gifts with which the dear God has blessed us, and we might well take care of them, instead of spoiling their beauty with grime and roughness.

Besides being sweetly clean, a woman's hand should have mental and moral meaning. We like best the strong, firm hand from whose clasp one secures sympathy, encouragement and friendship, the hand that shows energy and work as well as beauty, thoughtfulness as well as grace. There is nothing more exquisite than the soft, smooth pink finger nail on a woman's white hand. What a frightful thing to mar its loveliness by unkempt edges, raggedy flesh about it and, perish the thought, plain black grime under its fragile rosebud eyes.

"'Twas a hand
White, delicate, dimpled, warm, languid and bland.
The hand of a woman if often in youth
Somewhat rough, somewhat red, somewhat graceless, in truth;
Does its beauty refine, as its pulses grow calm,
Or as sorrow has crossed the life line in its palm?"

Care and scrupulous cleanliness are soon repaid in the toilet of the hands, and the busy housewife is included in this statement. Pure soap, which is not expensive, can be used instead of the ordinary laundry soap during the dish washing torments, while rubber gloves can be slipped on when the home is dusted and set to rights.

Chapped hands are often the result of poor circulation, and for that reason friction is beneficial.[xvi]

BEAUTY AND HAIR DRESSING OF 1912

The hands should be carefully dried after being bathed; they must not be exposed to sharp winds, and cold cream must be applied frequently. Occasionally some slight disturbance of the blood will cause an itching irritation.

It is the common and pernicious practice in America to cut the selvage skin which borders the nail inside and which is intended to protect it. Steel instruments should never be used under or around the finger nails. The very smoothest of these instruments is sharp enough to roughen the delicate under surface. It then attracts the dust and foreign matter because of this roughness, and more cleaning only makes it worse. The proper thing to use is an orangewood stick. The flesh about the nails must not be gouged and hacked and snipped.

The nails require a firm nail brush and soap at least once daily, and, after the tubbing, the flesh must be pushed back gently away from the nail. If this is done carefully every morning while the cuticle is soft from the action of the water, there will be no trouble with hangnails or roughened cuticle.

DIRECTIONS FOR MANICURING

The ordinary process of manicuring is as follows:

Soak the finger ends in a suds made of warm water and pure soap. Dry the fingers, pressing the selvage down all around. If little ends adhere to the nail, lift them up tenderly and carefully with an orangewood stick or possibly with the cuticle knife, although it is best never to use this at all, as it is likely to cause tiny white specks to form; cleanse the nails with the stick,

BEAUTY AND HAIR DRESSING OF 1912

then file them to an oval, going down not too far at the sides, and always filing toward the center.

Apply peroxide of hydrogen with the orangewood stick. If after the filing the under skin still shows a tiny white lining at the edges, remove this with beveling files of fine sandpaper. Hangnails should be dug away with a bit of pointed sandpaper or should be removed with the pointed scissors. Touch the finger nails with vaseline, then with nail powder,[xvii] and polish with a chamois skin buffer. There are other new polishes in cake form that combine the paste and the powder and these are much nicer than the old time method.[xviii] After the polishing, bathe the hands again in warm suds, dry carefully and give a final shine by rubbing in the moist palms of the hands.

White spots may be due to impaired circulation, gathering of natural fluids of the nail or misuse of instruments.[xix]

BEAUTY AND HAIR DRESSING OF 1912

BEAUTY AND HAIR DRESSING OF 1912

NOTES BY TALIA FELIX

[i] This is an old-fashioned belief. Modern research has shown hair loss to have many possible causes including malnutrition, hormone levels, skin disease and medicinal side-effects. Current research indicates that most scalps have sufficient blood supply to feed the hair follicles, even on those who have grown bald (as proven by the success of hair transplant surgery, which would fail if poor circulation were indeed the cause of the hair loss.) This belief is nevertheless held as popular folk-wisdom to this day.

[ii] The removal of actual dirt or other messes was understood to be the only reason for washing the hair in this era. The famous practice of a nightly "hundred strokes" with a natural-bristle hairbrush was used for the daily maintenance-cleaning of one's locks, for it brushed away lint and dandruff, and helped to distribute the oils of the hair in order to avoid a greasy appearance.

[iii] Current knowledge is that hair is colored with types of melanin: eumelanin for darker colors, pheomelanin for lighter shades. All humans have some pheomelanin in their hair color, and the concentration of eumelanin determines the darkness of the hair. Melanin is a pigment but it is a chemical not a mineral.

[iv] This refers to the practice of providing the wigmaker with a clipping of one's own hair to match with a wig or hairpiece.

[v] i.e. physical fitness.

BEAUTY AND HAIR DRESSING OF 1912

[vi] Bar soap like that used on the body or for laundry was used as shampoo, thus the need to dissolve it in advance. There were a handful of liquid shampoos available at this time, but these often amounted to little more than solutions of soap pre-dissolved in water and alcohol.

[vii] i.e. a shower attachment. Running water was had in many but not all homes by this era, but even among those who had such luxuries, the practice of showering to wash the hair was not the norm.

[viii] This appears to be based on the old medical belief that subjecting the skin to brief periods of coldness could permanently disrupt one's blood circulation. The instruction to use a warm towel and to massage the head would seem to be efforts to counteract the effects of the cold and wet.

[ix] The belief in the need to "exercise the scalp" again relates to theories of circulation as a means to improve hair growth. Modern thinking is that, while increasing circulation to the scalp is indeed beneficial, doing so by vigorous brushing can risk being too irritating to the skin and hair follicles and may actually cause greater harm than good.

[x] Hair tonics could be made in many different ways and for treating a variety of conditions. The most common ones of the era used irritating ingredients like spice oils and cantharides in order to stimulate the scalp. Other mixtures might be similar to modern conditioning or oil treatments, and still others might provide drying and mattifying properties for oily hair.

BEAUTY AND HAIR DRESSING OF 1912

A safe stimulating tonic can be made from 4 parts strongly brewed black tea, 1 part bay rum, 2 parts spirits of rosemary, and 1 part glycerin well mixed. - A gently moisturizing tonic can be prepared from 2 parts olive oil, 3 parts rubbing alcohol, 3 parts strong salt water, and 1 part spirits of lavender combined thoroughly.
In both cases the tonic should be shaken before use, and applied all over the scalp with fingers or with a toothbrush.

[xi] Skin foods were a type of lotion or moisturizer that were once popular. It was believed that they would plump (feed) the skin by its absorbing of their fatty ingredients.

[xii] Pure cornstarch or pure talcum powder are both period appropriate face powders. A very small amount of carmine or yellow ochre can be added in if a tint is desired, though plain white powder was very often used in this era.

[xiii] There were many different recipes for rouge, but they were most commonly colored with carmine. A period correct rouge can be made easily from plain carmine pigment dusted onto the cheeks with a brush. Cream rouge was also made by mixing the carmine into some kind of cream or solid fat.
Red was effectively the only color of rouge available, with pink shades occasionally made by diluting the red in a white colored base.

[xiv] "Greaseless cream" is the type of moisturizer we tend to be familiar with today. In 1912 it would be the same as the product known as vanishing cream. It was greaseless and vanishing in that it did not leave a slick oily layer behind on the skin, as did the more typical cold creams and skin foods.

BEAUTY AND HAIR DRESSING OF 1912

[xv] It was believed in this era that improved blood circulation and that "exercising" the facial muscles by rubbing them, could prevent and cure wrinkles – thus the notion that massage would aid in wrinkle reduction.

[xvi] Another old-fashioned belief relating to blood circulation.

[xvii] Nail powders were used to buff the fingernails and give a slight tint. Tin oxide alone was a common recipe for such powder, with the option of adding carmine for color or essential oils for scent. 200 parts zinc oxide colored with 2 parts carmine was another simple recipe.

[xviii] Cake nail buffing polish could be made by melting together (by weight) 5 parts white beeswax, 5 parts spermaceti and 10 parts paraffin. Into this hot liquid was beaten (by weight) 4 parts talc and 10 parts tin oxide, with continued beating and mashing until the mixture had stiffened and cooled.

[xix] These spots are now known to be caused by injury to the nail and occasionally by medical conditions. A persistent wives tale holds them to be caused by vitamin or mineral deficiency, but in such cases there would be other more severe symptoms present as well.

Made in the USA
San Bernardino, CA
06 June 2015